FIT BODY

BRYAN & STEPHANIE VIGNERY

Keep FIT BODY on your kitchen counter.

Let a healthy tip influence your better nutrition and activity choices today.

DAY ONE

The most important person who needs my care ... is me.

BENEFIT:

It is important to accept responsibility for taking care of ourselves. When we look and feel our best, we build up our self-confidence. And confidence can lead to being a better parent, spouse, neighbor, and friend. It leads to being more of the person we were created to be.

APPLICATION:

Get a journal and write a 60-item list of positives about yourself. If you find it challenging to come up with 60 items, ask the people around you what kinds of positive things they see in you. Add those things to the list. Keep the journal in a secure place. Go back and read it whenever you are feeling overwhelmed.

FIT BODY

If I don't have my health, I have nothing.

BENEFIT:

Throughout our life, we will have only one body. The body that seems invincible early on will be the same one with aches and pains in the middle years and the one with diminished function near the end. Treating our body right today can lessen those adverse effects of time well into our later years.

APPLICATION:

A good first step might be acknowledging that change is needed. Make a list of ten things about your health and well-being that you would like to see changed. From that list of ten, pick the three most essential items that you can begin to focus on first. Ask some tough questions and research the best answers. Today is the best time to start.

FIT BODY

Set goals! Be specific about what I want to accomplish and give myself a time frame to accomplish it in.

BENEFIT:

When we write something down, it becomes much clearer in our minds. *I will lose 30 pounds in 90 days.* We should tell someone what we have written. This creates a sense of accountability in us. Finally, let's do the work we need to do every day, believing that nothing will stop us from reaching your goal.

APPLICATION:

Take some time and begin to visualize yourself reaching your goal. How might you feel about the accomplishment? How might you feel about yourself? Then, speak your goal as though it has already been reached. *I have lost 30 pounds in 90 days.* Begin each activity associated with your goal by repeating your goal ten times out loud. Believe that it is as good as done.

DAY FOUR

Know and understand my 'why.' What is the why that will make me cry?

BENEFIT:

When the 'why' behind our goal is compelling, it can keep us going when the going gets tough. 'I am losing weight to look good on a cruise ship' probably won't cut it. But 'I am losing weight because heart disease runs in my family and I want to play with my grandkids' just might.

APPLICATION:

Write in your journal as many reasons as you can why you want to reach your goal. Then, identify the four most compelling reasons – your 'why.' Write out your real why on several notecards and place them where you will see them throughout the day – on your mirror, at your desk, on your dashboard, in the book you are currently reading, etc.

FIT BODY

Create a positive mental picture. Visualize it!

BENEFIT:

Are we still seeing ourselves reaching our goal? Can we see a clearer picture of what it looks like to accomplish it? Are we believing more and more that we can achieve what we want? What we think about and focus on tends to become our reality.

APPLICATION:

Take a few quiet moments to sit down and
visualize yourself reaching your goal. Then,
spend some time journaling how it might feel
to accomplish it. Write it and rewrite it. Read
it and reread it. Keep your journal in front of
you daily.

DAY 5

DAY SIX

Clear my mind of self-doubt. My mindset is key.

BENEFIT:

A lot of people can easily see the negative. So, for them, here is a list of things we can't do. We can't go there. We can't buy into negative beliefs or counterproductive self-talk. We can't create and maintain harmful environments. We can't spend all our time around negative influences. And we can't wait to be rid of the "can't do" way of living which others can easily see.

APPLICATION:

Few people can consistently believe the positive. So, for you, here is a list of things you can believe about yourself. I am strong. I am disciplined. I am able to make good choices in my life. I am able to create good daily habits. I am consistent. I am healthy. I am able to do anything I set my mind to do. Write these "I am" statements, and some of your own, in your journal.

DAY 6

FIT BODY

DAY SEVEN

Embrace the challenge and equip myself for it. Take things one day at a time.

BENEFIT:

Today is the only day that we can begin to do something differently. Within weeks, that change can become a habit. More changes and better habits later, a new way develops, until the process becomes a healthy lifestyle over time. And just think; it all started with today.

APPLICATION:

You have probably heard that it takes 21 days to establish a new habit. I challenge you to come up with five simple things you could do today that will lead to your better health. Then, choose one to focus on for the next 21 days. (Don't worry. You will choose each of the other four as time goes on.) Remember, it takes healthy daily habits to create lifestyle results.

DAY 7

FIT BODY

DAY EIGHT

Stay on track. Remember that consistency plus discipline equals results.

BENEFIT:

Consistency will get us there; discipline will keep us there, even if the process is less than perfect. So what should a person do if they get off track? Get back on. Keep pressing forward. The desired result is still achievable. There is something truly amazing about failing; we can fail backward or fail forward. The choice is ours.

APPLICATION:

Backup plans can save the day when things don't go perfectly, and you are tempted to give up. For example, keep a bag with workout clothes and shoes in your car, in case you run out of time to pack a bag. Doing little things like this will help keep you on track toward your goal. Now, what backup plan can you think of which might help you stay on track?

FIT BODY

Prove to myself that I can do it. Actions speak louder than words.

BENEFIT:

We will not have a fit body until we have a fit mind. Change doesn't always equal growth, but growth always equals change. It's not about proving something to someone else; it's about proving to ourselves that we can do it. No one can take care of us but us. Now, let's stop talking about it and go do it.

APPLICATION:

It is make-it-happen time. Consider joining a gym or clearing a space at home for your workouts. Consider hiring a trainer or meeting with an accountability partner. Put all of your planned workouts for the month on a paper calendar and on your phone, as well. Checkmark your calendar every time you complete a scheduled workout. This will help keep you accountable and stay motivated.

FIT BODY

*Engage an accountability partner or coach—
someone I trust, who will push me beyond
my comfort zone.*

BENEFIT:

We can be a highly disciplined person, but
most people are not self-motivated enough
to do something truly out of their comfort
zone. It is much easier to meet someone
for a workout than it is to go and workout by
ourselves.

APPLICATION:

If you are struggling with self-discipline and could use some motivation, I strongly encourage you to reach out and invite someone to join you. Who knows; that person might be feeling something similar. By having the confidence to step out and ask for help, you could be helping someone else in your shoes.

DAY 10

FIT BODY

DAY ELEVEN

Stay active on a daily basis.

BENEFIT:

There are certainly health benefits of staying physically active. But while we work toward having a fit body, we should also pursue a fit spirit and a fit mind. Each of these areas can have a positive effect on the other two. Spending time every day actively focused on these three areas goes a long way toward developing a well-balanced life.

APPLICATION:

Create an action plan for the week. Make a list of things that would help you stay active spiritually, personally, and physically. Make it a list of things you enjoy doing. It will be much easier to stick with it. Stay consistent, and you will be amazed at how much better you will feel when you create this time in your daily routine.

DAY TWELVE

Cardio, Cardio, Cardio

BENEFIT:

Cardio (aerobic exercise) is one of the best things we can do for mental, emotional, and physical health. It builds strength and endurance, burns calories and fat, and helps with weight loss. It is particularly healthy for reducing belly fat, which builds up around our organs. Cardio activity is most beneficial when done for 20 minutes at a steady pace. Adding weights to our cardio workout is also beneficial.

APPLICATION:

Make it a point to do your cardio workout
for at least 20 minutes. If that is too difficult
at first, go for as long as you can, then add
a minute or two on the following days. If 20
minutes of steady-pace cardio is no problem
for you, I will challenge you to change things
up and try an interval cardio workout this
week or another type of cardio workout that
is different than what you have been doing.

DAY 12

FIT BODY

FIT BODY

DAY THIRTEEN

*Incorporate weights or resistance training
into my workout. Use dumbbells and
barbells, resistance bands, and weighted
exercise balls.*

BENEFIT:

Lifting weights is one of the best things we
can do for body composition and strength.
Resistance training has profound effects
on many areas of the body. The addition of
weights or resistance to our workout helps
build muscle, and it doesn't take a lot to see
a difference. The more muscle we build, the
more fat we will burn.

APPLICATION:

Develop a workout plan before you start. This will help you have better workouts and keep you on track. Set a goal to start lifting one to three times a week, whether at a gym or at home. If your goal is to lean out, do more reps with less weight. To build muscle, do fewer reps with heavier weight. The most important thing, of course, is to start. I know you will be glad you did.

DAY FOURTEEN

It's 80% nutrition; 20% my workout.

BENEFIT:

The food we put in our body is the fuel that makes it work. In most cases, the reflection we see in the mirror is a result of the quality of the fuel we have put into our body and the quality of the work we have done to burn it, compounded over time. The good news is that we can change a poor reflection by feeding our body the fuel it really needs and burning that fuel by actively working out—consistently.

FIT BODY

APPLICATION:

Clear out your pantry and refrigerator of junk food items and replace them with the nutrition your body needs. (You will not only be addressing your own health but the health of your loved ones as well.) Be intentional about what you put in your mouth. Focus on greens, proteins, good carbohydrates, and good fats. Give yourself smaller portion sizes throughout the day. Eat when you are hungry, but stop before you get too full. Keep the carb intake lower at night. And be consistent with your workouts.

DAY FIFTEEN

Water, water, water. I have to stay hydrated.

BENEFIT:

Being properly hydrated has many benefits, including increased energy and a boost in brainpower. Adding lemon juice to 8 ounces of water first thing in the morning helps kick start our metabolism, relieves dehydration, stimulates the digestive system, and helps with weight loss. Lemon water in the evening detoxes the colon, boosts the immune system, helps with heartburn, and helps reduce inflammation.

APPLICATION:

We should be drinking no less than 64 fluid ounces of water each day, which is eight 8 oz. glasses. A more proper formula is "between half an ounce and a full ounce of water for each pound you weigh." I would suggest getting yourself a water jug. It will help you keep better track of how much water you are drinking. Pour your water into a cup with a straw and add lemon for taste.

DAY SIXTEEN

Don't forget good, healthy snacking.

BENEFIT:

Some people have a misconception that snacking is bad. When we snack on the right kinds of food, it is actually a very healthy thing to do. One or two snacks at the proper time of the day can keep our metabolism working for us and help keep us from feeling too hungry, which is why we often overeat at mealtime.

APPLICATION:

If you only eat meals and tend to overeat when you do, try incorporating a mid-morning or mid-afternoon snack into your day (maybe veggies with hummus, a handful of almonds, or a tuna packet). If time tends to get away from you during your busy day, try setting the alarm to remind yourself to snack. If you already eat a snack or two but aren't seeing the results you desire, take a look at what you are snacking on. When all else fails, there's always protein.

DAY SEVENTEEN

Make protein a part of every meal and snack.

BENEFIT:

High protein intake can boost our metabolism and help us build lean muscle. At the same time, it keeps us more sustained and feeling full, so we are not continually feeling hungry. It will help reduce our cravings, so we don't end up going to foods that are not as healthy for us. Eating protein with carbohydrates helps balance out the sugars in the carbs.

APPLICATION:

Eat a small portion of protein with every meal. Because protein is more sustaining and keeps you feeling fuller longer, eat the protein on your plate before anything else. That way, you are sure to get the protein you need. If you find that you are still hungry, the best thing to do is to increase your protein and fibrous veggies without eating more carbohydrates and fats. Also keep in mind, though, that still feeling hungry after eating may be an indication of dehydration.

DAY 17

DAY EIGHTEEN

Be watchful of fruit when it comes to sugar.

BENEFIT:

We shouldn't think that fruit is bad for us,
but rather keep in mind that it is sugar. If our
goal is to lose weight or lean out, it is best to
keep the sugars low.

APPLICATION:

When you eat fruit, and you're trying to keep sugar intake lower, any type of berries is your best choice. Also, when you eat a piece of fruit, it is best to balance out the sugars with a protein, especially pre- and post-workout. Morning time is best for fruit intake. Minimize fruit intake at night.

DAY NINETEEN

Watch my sugar and sodium intake.

BENEFIT:

Sugar and sodium can hurt us more than help us. The more we eat sugar, the more we crave it, and if we are not burning it off, our body will store it. There are a lot of hidden sugars in foods. Key words to look for on the food labels are sucrose, lactose, maltose, sorbitol, dextrose, fructose, glucose, and high fructose corn syrup. Too much sodium causes us to retain water weight. Drinking more water is the best way to flush out the extra water weight.

APPLICATION:

Carbohydrates are another form of sugar. Some carbs are higher in sugar than others. "Good carbs" include brown rice, oatmeal (not instant), sweet potatoes, and quinoa. "Bad carbs" include potato chips, candy bars, and soda pop. It's best to focus more on good carbs, but that doesn't mean you can't have bad carbs once in a while. You want good carbs more consistently than bad. If you have a sugar addiction, go 21 days with low sugar intake. Your body will begin detoxing from sugar, and you will find that your body will not crave it as much.

FIT BODY

Beware of juices and alcohol. Too much of either can hinder my weight loss.

BENEFIT:

If we are not getting results as quickly as we desire, we should take a look at what we are drinking. Juices and alcohol can negatively impact our weight loss. Alcohol slows the metabolism down, which means we will store more fat. If we are going to drink, red wine is a much better option than margaritas and daiquiris, which are loaded with sugar. A good philosophy is that we can never go wrong with drinking water.

APPLICATION:

Although the comments about alcohol don't apply if you are a non-drinker, you still need to be mindful of sodas, juices, and other sugary drinks. If these kinds of drinks are a downfall to you, cut your intake in half.

If you do drink and it is every night or every other night, cut your intake in half immediately. You should start to feel better and see your body beginning to respond. You may even work yourself down to only having alcohol during a cheat meal — everything in moderation.

DAY TWENTY-ONE

Relaxed Meals

BENEFIT:

A relaxed meal has its place, but we shouldn't see it as a reward for all the hard work we have done. Better health and fitness are rewards for that. However, a relaxed meal can shock the body and help reset our metabolism. Although it is okay to have slices of pizza and a bowl of ice cream (without any guilt) anytime, it may be best to play our 'relaxed meal card' at times like family gatherings, birthday parties, a night out with friends, etc.

APPLICATION:

I challenge you to do one—and only one—relaxed meal this week. I do mine on the 6th or 7th day. Because your body's metabolism has been high throughout the week, your relaxed meal will burn off a lot quicker.
The key is to jump back on board with your health plan the next day. Oh! And don't be surprised if you are a little swollen from taking-in more sodium than you are used to. Drinking a little extra water will flush out those toxins.

Dining Out

BENEFIT:

Sometimes, our relaxed meal will be dinner at a restaurant. But, dinner out can also be within our normal healthy routine if we make good choices. A salad loaded with veggies is a great option. If we make sure the dressing is on the side, we can control how much of it we eat. Vinaigrettes are better than creamy dressings. We can save hundreds of calories by dipping our fork into the dressing. It is not a good idea to eat out more than once a week.

FIT BODY

APPLICATION:

If eating out is a temptation for you, try
this strategy. Research moderately-priced,
healthy restaurant choices in your area.
What do others on a health journey suggest?
Go out on your "relaxed day," but set your
mind that your choices will reflect and
respect your healthy meals throughout the
week. Choose a salad with dressing on the
side. Choose chicken or beef without bread
(no bun or half the bun if it is a sandwich).
Or even make it a lettuce wrap. And instead
of French fries, choose raw or steamed
veggies.

DAY 22

FIT BODY

DAY TWENTY-THREE

Not all carbohydrates are bad; some are healthy.

BENEFIT:

A healthy lifestyle will always be based on a proper balance of all of the food groups. Our body needs lean proteins, healthy fats, and complex carbohydrates. Someone who doesn't work out much may not need as many carbs as someone who works out every day, and everyone's body is different. However, we need good carbs and healthy fats for fuel and energy. Remember; add a protein if we need to balance the sugars.

APPLICATION:

One of the best time options for eating good carbs and protein is right after your workout. It helps refuel your muscles so they can burn fat. An excellent choice would be a protein shake with almond milk and fresh berries. If you don't like shakes, try preparing one egg with two additional egg whites and fresh berries on the side. Or scramble cooked sweet potatoes with your eggs, and add just a pinch of salt and pepper for extra taste.

DAY 23

DAY TWENTY-FOUR

Prepare my meals ahead of time.

BENEFIT:

Prepping our meals in advance is one of the most important things we can do when we are working to reach any type of health goal. Food prep is a time-saver throughout our week, and it puts healthy options at our fingertips if we are hit with an urge to 'raid the fridge.' It takes a good amount of time to prep a week's worth of meals, so let's make sure we dedicate a part of our weekend schedule to it.

APPLICATION:

If preparing your meals ahead of time is new to you, try this. Set aside a couple of hours, maybe on Sunday afternoon, to prepare lunches for the next few days (especially if you work outside the home). Prepare two or three pieces of chicken. Cook some brown rice and sweet potatoes, and cut up some veggies and lettuce. Keep the food in the refrigerator or a small cooler until you are ready to warm it up and eat it.

DAY 24

FIT BODY

DAY TWENTY-FIVE

Stress is common to everyone. I will learn to handle mine well.

BENEFIT:

Stress offers no physical benefits, but we will never be able to remove it completely from our lives. So it is important that we learn to manage stress properly to decrease its negative effects on our body. When we 'stress out,' our body releases the hormone cortisol, which makes it more difficult to lose belly fat. There may be other reasons why we have trouble losing inches around our midsection, but stress is a factor that we cannot overlook.

APPLICATION:

Because short, quicks breaths are why cortisol is released, the most important thing you can do to combat the effects of stress is to take long, deep breaths. This also helps to relax you. Then, you should write down in a journal or notebook what it is that is causing the stress. (Reading a few encouraging pages of Fit Spirit or Fit Mind might also help.) When stress happens quickly, just think: Stop, Breathe, Pray, Release.

DAY TWENTY-SIX

The most effective technique to prevent injury is stretching.

BENEFIT:

Stretching helps keep us flexible and injury-free. It should be done for 5-10 minutes before and after each workout. Also, stretch before every strenuous activity in our everyday life (helping someone move, etc.). Stretching just after getting out of bed is also beneficial. When the whole idea of it is new to someone, it is a good idea to take a yoga class or watch a video. It is a great way to learn solid stretching routines.

APPLICATION:

Whether you are currently working out or not, make it your goal to stretch three to five times this week. Even if you are not used to it, it is important to start. If you already stretch on a regular basis, work toward stretching 20-30 minutes each time.

DAY 26

DAY TWENTY-SEVEN

Create a healthy lifestyle with my whole family.

BENEFIT:

When we are a good example of a healthy lifestyle—with a clearer mind, more energy, and less stress—we are showing our children that, they too, can make good choices in their lives, which can then have a positive effect on our grandchildren's generation as well. So, let's focus on eating healthy meals and engaging in positive activities together. We just might find ourselves staying on track much better than we used to.

APPLICATION:

This week, go through your cabinets and get rid of the overabundance of processed foods. Your kids don't have to go 'all-organic' on Day One, but sugar—especially high fructose corn syrup—has got to be the first to go. Eating less sugar produces fewer cravings for sugar, and not having it in the house makes it less of a temptation. Another rule of thumb; foods with fewer ingredients are better.

DAY TWENTY-EIGHT

Sleep is paramount for my health.

BENEFIT:

The importance of getting enough quality sleep cannot be overstated. One of the most substantial risk factors for weight gain and obesity is lack of sleep. Getting enough sleep is as important, if not more so, as nutrition and staying active. Without a consistent schedule for nighttime sleeping, it is much more challenging for us to metabolize food, manage stress levels, and have enough energy for a proper workout.

APPLICATION:

Everyone is different when it comes to how much sleep they need. If you don't already know how much you need, make it a priority to research it for yourself. When you know, set a schedule if you have difficulty falling asleep, try these suggestions: just before you get into bed, do some stretching, write in a journal for 15 minutes, or spend time in prayer; drink decaffeinated herbal tea with honey; or take a bath with lavender in the water.

DAY 28

FIT BODY

DAY TWENTY-NINE

Probiotics, Vitamins, Minerals, and Omega-3 Fatty Acids

BENEFIT:

Knowing the food groups, knowing the nutrients that are found within those food groups, and knowing the proper amounts of those nutrients that our body needs will help us to help our body work the way it was designed to. Even still, there may be a need to supplement some vitamins and minerals, or Omega-3 oils, or probiotics.

APPLICATION:

My challenge for you today is to do some research into a good multivitamin and a good probiotic supplement and begin taking them as soon as you can. This will help to fill in the gaps in your nutrient intake. In addition to this, commit to learning more about food groups and what it would take to get the proper amounts of the nutrients your body needs.

DAY 29

FIT BODY

FIT BODY

DAY THIRTY

I will keep a 'gratitude list.'

BENEFIT:

It is too easy for us to see the negative that goes on around us and inside us. Keeping a list of the things we are thankful for, and reading through it when we need to, can help us focus on the blessings in our life. Our mindset will change for the better when we focus on the positive.

APPLICATION:

Get a journal or a notebook, and keep it with you as often as you can. For 21 days in a row (you are creating a new habit here), write down five things you are grateful for. Push yourself to think 'outside the box.' Someone once said, "If you had to list 200 blessings that you are truly thankful for, I guarantee that #200 would be a great one. Because more thought went into that one than all the others." Maybe you should call this a "Blessing List."

DAY THIRTY-ONE

Don't forget about water!

BENEFIT:

There is no benefit to being dehydrated, so understanding the necessity of water is very, very important. When we are dehydrated, we are in survival mode, instead of thriving as we should be. Yet, we tend to adapt to our own dryness. By the time we feel thirsty, we are already dehydrated. It affects our mood, our attentiveness, and fine-motor coordination. If we do not take in water, even our ability to perceive properly can be negatively affected.

Jesus said, "Everyone who drinks
from this water will get thirsty again.
But whoever drinks from the water
that I will give him will never get thirsty
again. In fact, the water I will give him will
become a well of water springing up in him
for eternal life."

(John 4:13–14 CSB)

DAY 31

FIT BODY